*The Basics Series*
*For Hospital-Based Group Leaders*

AF811502

# Hospital-Based Medical Group Mergers, Acquisitions and Alternatives

MARK F. WEISS

Published by The Mark F. Weiss Law Firm, a Professional Corporation
1227 De La Vina Street
Santa Barbara, CA 93101
310-843-2800



---



---

For information about Mark F. Weiss's services and speaking, please call 310-843-2800 or email request@advisorylawgroup.com. Free articles, videos, podcasts and the archive of the Advisory e-Alert, our electronic newsletter, are available at www.advisorylawgroup.com.

Visit www.advisorylawgroup.com to subscribe to our complimentary monthly e-Alert and to follow the link to Mark's frequently updated Wisdom. Applied. blog.

ISBN:0692387951
ISBN-13:9780692387955

# CONTENTS

# ABOUT THE AUTHOR

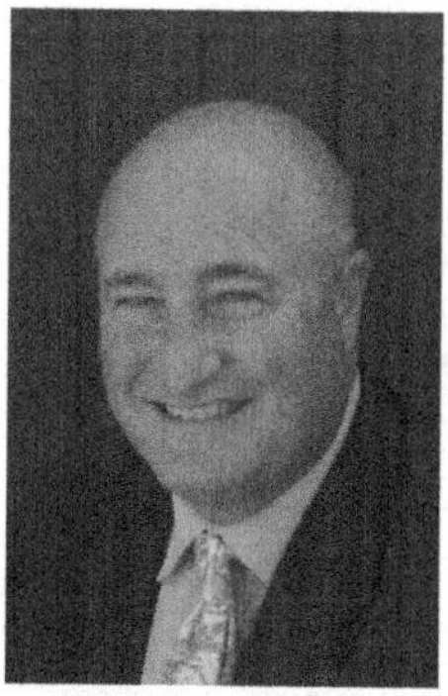

Mark F. Weiss is an expert on the legal and business issues affecting medical groups, entrepreneurial physicians, and healthcare businesses.

Mr. Weiss advises clients nationally on achieving their goals, maximizing their profits and managing their risk of loss.

Lawyers often view the world though a microscope trained to see the minutia of the "legal" issue and, as a result, ignore virtually everything else. As a result, they preach a purely "legal solution" that, quite often, is worthless in terms of any practical benefit for you.

Mr. Weiss views the world differently: He and his firm, The Mark F. Weiss Law Firm, operate on the same entrepreneurial level as do you. He understands that legal issues are intertwined with your business issues and cannot be separated. He understands that psychological and political issues often transcend the obvious issues.

Mr. Weiss is a frequent speaker and the author of more than 200 articles on issues affecting healthcare providers. From 2002 through 2013, he held an appointment as a clinical assistant professor at USC's Keck School of Medicine.

Contact Mr. Weiss by email at markweiss@advisorylawgroup.com or by phone at 310-843-2800.

# INTRODUCTION

As I write this, a combination of factors is causing acceleration in the market for hospital-based medical group mergers and acquisitions.

Obamacare is shifting economic power to hospitals.

Many physicians, especially those who are not particularly entrepreneurial, are moving to hospital employment or otherwise being "aligned," resulting in changing referral patters.

Private equity money has entered the market.

Practices that could never, or barely, have been sold ten years ago, are now, in some cases, valued at high multiples of earnings.

As you might expect, some hospital-based group leaders see the potential for a sale as a panacea. They fear that reimbursement may fall, and their hospital-contracts might be lost. So shift, they think, that risk to someone else and pocket some profit to boot.

Others see opportunity in this market through an entirely different lens. They see tremendous advantage in remaining independent or in structuring their own ventures.

Finally, another subset is confused and worried about the future and lacks the structure to take any action at all.

But no matter where you fall in that continuum, this book is aimed at providing both medical group leaders and the physician owners of those groups with a basic understanding of hospital-based group acquisitions and, importantly, the alternatives.

# PART ONE

## Background: Market Realities -- Relationship Between Groups And Hospitals

# CHAPTER 1

## What Maintains The Relationship Between A Hospital-Based Physician Group And A Hospital? And, What Disrupts It . . . *Really*?

For all the talk of a healthcare system, the relationship between hospitals and hospital-based groups is becoming even more of a *market.*

In fact, it's not all that different from the market for those in the grocery market business.

We've got independent markets. We've got giant chains like Safeway (which is also Vons, Randall's, Tom Thumb, and Carr's and even more), Kroger and Publix. We've got very high end markets such as Gelson's in Southern California or Whole Foods. And we've got little corner convenience markets.

Safeway and Kroger and Publix and the other giant chains haven't put Trader Joes out of business. No more so than large hospitals have put all surgeon owned specialty hospitals or ambulatory surgery centers out of business.

So, in this market, what maintains the relationship between the incumbent hospital-based physician group and a hospital? And, what disrupts it?

Although it may not appear as such at first, this is an extremely important bit of background information in connection with the notion of mergers and acquisitions and other alternatives.

After all, if your group is going to be acquired, what exactly is being acquired if it's not the relationship between your group and the hospitals and the other facilities at which you provide services?

And, if you're going to be engaging in any of the alternatives I'll discuss later in the book, you'd better be damn sure you understand what causes stickiness in terms of the relationship between your group and the facility or facilities at which it provides services.

For the most part, the world still is the incumbent group's oyster. Incumbent groups are still largely in charge of their own destiny. Note that I said largely, not completely, in charge. No one is ever completely in charge in terms of contracting with someone else.

So, to a very large extent, the group with the contract is still largely in the position to keep it. That is, until they screw things up and cause it to be lost.

How do they screw things up? Generally, by pissing off the customer.

But that leads to the age-old hospital-based group question: Who is the customer?

*Who Is The Customer?*

Traditionally, hospital-based groups are seen as having multiple types of customers:

1. Patients.
2. Referring physicians such as those ordering imaging studies from radiologists, or surgeons as to anesthesiologists.
3. The hospital itself, from hospital staff members with whom you work on a day-to-day basis all the way up to the greater relationship with hospital administration.

*Some Customers Are More Equal*

Although all three categories describe customers, the truth is that some customers are more equal that others. And, of course, as anyone with experience working on the relationship between hospital–based groups and hospitals knows for certain, the hospital itself is the most important customer.

Don't get me wrong, great patient care is what healthcare is all about.

However, when we're talking about relationship in the context of this book, we're talking about the relationship between your group and the hospital and its administration.

Sure, patient complaints get back to the issue of how groups service the hospital.

And yes, referring physician complaints which get back to hospital administration impact that evaluation of how a group services the hospital.

The key here is that the relationship with hospital administration is central. After all, it's through the hospital administration that the hospital either enters into, or doesn't enter into, the contract with your group.

*Complaints*

When things begin to go awry between hospitals and groups, these are the sort of complaints that hospitals levy:

1. Your group has no leadership.
2. Your group is dysfunctional.
3. We pay you too high of a stipend – "You're too expensive."
4. There's no/poor alignment between your group and the hospital's interests:
    - Your group is not responsive to our valid complaints.
    - Your group never creates new value for the hospital (you're not proactive).
    - Your group refuses to change with the times.

And, it's even worse than that in that these same issues are the "selling points" that aggressive groups of all sorts – not just the true groups, but also contract management companies and staffing services – use to try to disrupt the relationship between the hospital and the incumbent group.

*Switching Costs*

Perhaps the greatest benefit to an incumbent group is the fact that, for the hospitals they contract with, there's a significant cost to switching groups. That cost can be measured in time, in money, and in liability.

Switching often causes turmoil within the hospital.

Generally speaking, the physician members of the former group were on staff for many years, in some cases for many decades. Those familiar faces are now gone. Or worse, they are still there but about to lose their staff privileges, and they are not going without making a last stand, or, at least, a big stink.

Other contract holders, from other hospital-based groups to office–based physicians who hold medical directorships and other contracts, become concerned that the hospital will terminate their agreements, too.

As things progress and sometimes snowball, mid-level hospital administrators who participated in the decision to terminate the incumbent group often find themselves terminated as higher-level administrators run for cover – after all, someone has to be blamed.

There's also the risk of potential litigation. The hospital may have staged a fictitious request for proposal process in order to project a patina of fairness while, in actuality, the decision had already been made not to award a renewal contract to the incumbent group. They were lured into participating but stood no chance of getting the contract – they were defrauded.

The change may result in upsetting and even driving away referring physicians. And, in some cases, switching results in a crisis in terms of staffing – the new group promised a lot but delivers a little, what I call as Promise-Delivery Gap™.

So you can see that in light of these potential costs, there generally has to be something seriously wrong with the incumbent group or with its performance or with its relationship with the hospital and hospital administration to cause the hospital to switch.

That's why I state above that deals are generally the incumbent group's to lose. Sure, there are outlier events, in which little is wrong but the hospital administrator just pulls the trigger, but that can be a very expensive "shot."

So while those outliers exist, generally, critical mass must be reached in terms of factors that are either negative on the part of the incumbent group or extremely positive on the part of a potential new group, before the seesaw flips, destroying the incumbent group's leverage.

But, like a butcher who uses his finger to give a little bit of tilt to the scale, although the incumbent group still controls most of what's weighting this seesaw, you can be certain that competitors are attempting to tilt it the other way.

# CHAPTER 2

## How Are Your Competitors Competing?

In the 1980's most hospital-based groups didn't compete for anything. They just existed. If they were prescient enough to enter into a contract with the hospital at which they worked, they generally refused to consider competing beyond its four walls. After all, the guys working at the hospital down the road or across town were "colleagues," and, they thought, colleagues just don't compete with colleagues.

Unfortunately, not much has changed for the majority of groups. They still just are. It's just that they're no longer safe from mistaken beliefs about competition.

So, the real generational difference is that a minority of groups, a significant minority at that, joined by contract management companies and staffing services, is competing aggressively for hospital contracts and even system wide contracts.

In order to better understand how your competitors are competing, it helps to first understand *who* is competing. And the best way to start that process is to break these competitors down into categories.

3. No real business infrastructure.

Defensive groups usually lack any real business structure.

They sometimes have elected or institutionalized leaders, but they generally run on consensus, which means they are unfocused.

In the words of G.K. Chesterton, "I've searched all the parks in all the cities and found no statues of committees."

And they usually outsource all business services to a billing service. Note that outsourcing these back office functions is not necessarily a bad thing if the group has strong leadership that is willing to set the course for the group's future and to then see it through, even if that course initially fails.

4. Provide Services At One Hospital Only.

If a hospital-based group is defined by the existence of a single hospital contract, once that contract is lost, the group no longer has any reason to exist. On a very real level, the group really doesn't operate a *business*; it simply operates a *service* for that hospital.

The mere fact that the hospital's administration knows that weakness shifts incredible negotiating power to the facility: They know that they have you over a barrel. If they don't renew your exclusive contract, you are out of business.

5. Everything Is A Cost.

And now the mother of all underlying issues: Defensive groups tend to be too cheap to invest in themselves. To a defensive group, nothing is an investment – everything is a cost.

The driving motive for these groups is usually the current, regular and ongoing distribution of as much cash to the group's owner-physicians as is possible. As a result, anything, yes *anything*, that reduces that cash flow is highly suspect. "Do we really need to buy it? Can we get it for less? Let's put it off until next month or next quarter or next year."

So, those who have no problem spending $125,000 on a Porsche won't invest $10,000 in their group's future.

That thinking is like an anchor on a group's future: it pulls it down into the abyss of failure.

Amateurs view expenses as costs. Professionals view them as investments.

6. Many In No Position To Attract A Real Buyer.

Assuming for a moment that a defensive group is interested in exploring a sale to a national group or other aggregator, many defensive groups are not in any credible position to attract such a buyer.

Due to their defensive posture, they are usually too small to be an interesting acquisition target. They expended their efforts and energy toward defending their business, not toward growing it. This generally results in a smaller group, both in terms of providers and in terms of the number of facilities served.

And, when it comes to the one hospital or perhaps one hospital and a few surgery centers at which they provide services, they tend to be dependent on stipend support.

Many potential buyers, though not all, view heavy dependence on stipend support to be a large negative: What will happen to the group and its ability to both recruit, retain and remit a profit to its new owner if the stipend is cut? That's often enough to cause many significant buyers to end discussions with the group.

Last, it's usually the case that defensive groups have poor reimbursing payor contracts. They've simply not devoted the time and effort to negotiate higher rates. And, usually being held hostage in a sense by the one hospital contact they hold, they fear that pushing third party payors for increases will detrimentally impact their hospital relationship and, therefore, terminate their business existence.

Crummy reimbursement leads to low compensation. As you'll learn later in this book, buyers generally buy groups based on a multiple of a portion of cash flow. The remaining portion of cash must be sufficient to recruit and retain at the group level because it's the source of the funds used for compensation.

Most defensive groups' exclusive contracts, and physicians, are targets for *predatory groups*; these defensive groups are not targets for buyers that are willing to pay for their practices. Some defensive groups might be able to hang on due to fact that they are located at hospitals that are not attractive targets. Otherwise, their only hope for a long term future is to become a strategic group.

*Local – Strategic*

Let's turn our attention to the other category of local groups, those that are strategic.

By observation, this is a significantly smaller subset of local groups.

Here are some of the common characteristics of groups that fall into this segment.

1. <u>They Have Reached Critical Mass</u>.

There's no hard and fast number, and a strategic focus is, at its heart, based on both mindset and movement, but groups that are strategic tend to have developed into a significant size.

Note that size alone is not an indicator of strategic development, it's only a factor that might indicate the presence of a strategic mindset.

For example, a group that provides services at one large hospital only, that is, it doesn't provide service at any other facilities of any kind, might have over 100 members due to the sheer size of the facility served. At the same time, that group is likely completely defensive in its focus.

2. They Work At Multiple Hospitals.

Strategic groups have developed a real business; they're not simply providing a service *to* a hospital. They've grown their business so that their providers work at multiple hospitals and other facilities.

In fact, if their strategic mindset is well developed, they view themselves as being in business *with* the facilities they serve.

I can't stress how important working at multiple facilities is for a hospital-based group. It's what distinguishes a real business from a simple service.

If all your group does is provide service to one hospital, even to one hospital and one or two small surgery centers or similar facilities, then if the hospital terminates your contract, your group will no longer have any reason to exist.

I can guaranty you that in that situation, the administrator of the hospital, if he or she is worth anything, will know that the hospital holds the keys to your future in its hands. How tight they squeeze you is up to them.

I see this time and time again with weak groups. They are living on borrowed time. Local groups that are strategic, and all large groups, understand this lesson: The don't let themselves fall prey to their own failure to project their business power *beyond* one or even two or three major facilities.

3. They Likely Have A Real Business Infrastructure

Strategic local groups are run as actual businesses, not simply as clubs. As such, it's highly likely that they have a significant business infrastructure.

They or may not operate their own, in-house billing and collection operation, but they certainly have a physician CEO or managing partner who devotes significant time and effort to managing the group's business and, perhaps, an executive director, whether titled a business manager, chief operating officer, or by some other designation.

Importantly, the physician leaders of the group are allowed time away from their clinical duties in order to make time for management activities. Management isn't something that squeezed in at midnight or after hours. If the managing partner can't attend a meeting with, for example, the group's accounting firm at 2:00 p.m. upon a few day's notice, the group is an amateur, not strategic. The same goes for groups that regularly hold their meetings over dinner or in the evening or on weekends – it's a gigantic sign of amateur status.

Hand in hand with allowing the leaders, both physician and lay, to manage, a strategic group understands that not every effort, every initiative, every plan will be successful. Failure in medical *practice* can mean fatal – as in fatal for the patient and for your career. Failure in business is *expected*; you just re-group, having learned a lesson from the failure, and you keep on going. Strategic groups let their leaders fail forward, faster.

And, strategic groups pay their leaders for their leadership efforts. No one with serious leadership skills is going to take time away from patient care – if that is the only measure of performance that comes with pay – to attend a meeting. If your group doesn't understand this, if it thinks it's a good business decision to "save" $300,000 on leadership pay at the cost of its entire future, then lobby fast for a change and, failing its accomplishment, look fast for a new job.

4. They Invest In Themselves

Unlike defensive groups that view everything as a cost to be avoided, strategic local groups understand the value of making an investment. And, they understand that their best investment is in themselves.

Other groups run like vending machines: Their efforts, like soft drinks and snacks, are dispensed to patients. And the money deposited into it is emptied out on a regular basis, certainly zeroed out by year end.

Strategic group leaders understand that the best way to increase the group's members' incomes over the long haul is to invest in the protection of the group's business interests and in the expansion of the group's business interests. Accordingly, they "bank" cash within the group, establish reserves for their growth initiatives, and invest in outside advice, importing the expertise that the group lacks. They know that even $500,000 isn't the change a $20,000,000 a year group would leave behind in the cushions when it gets up from the couch.

As I mentioned above, amateurs view expenses as costs; professionals view them as investments: *investments in themselves.*

5. Market Gravitas

As a direct result of investing in themselves, in growing with the facilities they already serve, and in pushing to expand to other local facilities, strategic local groups develop what I call market gravitas.

That is, they become big enough for other facilities to take them seriously. This greases their efforts at further expansion. It creates marketing, and growth, momentum.

Because they are big enough and because they are seen as significant players in the market, they gain from the social proof of their past and current success. When they approach a new facility they are a known quantity with a known quality.

This same gravitas carries over to make strategic groups more attractive candidates for a potential acquisition. It also makes them potential acquirers and attractive deal partners for other groups, both strategic and defensive.

*Segmenting Large Groups*

Just as we segmented local groups into defensive and strategic, we can sort large groups into subcategories, too.

For our purposes, let's look at them in several ways.

First, we can segment them as predatory versus symbiotic. Second, we can segment them into single specialty versus multispecialty. And third, we can look at large groups and sort them in terms of their strategic vision.

*Large – Predatory*

With some exception, large predatory groups have a primary strategy that doesn't center on *buying* local groups; their primary strategy is to seek hospital contracts directly.

In other words, they don't buy, they take.

They do this in ways unfamiliar to all but the most sophisticated local groups: they telemarket, they send direct mail, they respond to RFPs, they do on-site visits (read that as the fact that they have salespeople who make direct contact with hospital administrators), and they have professional marketing and sales staff.

Frankly, I use the word "predatory" in order to get your attention. I could just as easily say "organically growing" – in other words these groups focus, in varying degrees, on picking up business not by acquiring local groups but, rather, by selling directly into hospitals.

Note that being predatory isn't like being pregnant: you can be a little bit or a lotta bit predatory. You can buy groups, on the one hand, and still market directly to hospitals, on the other.

*Large – Symbiotic*

As to the segment that I describe as large and symbiotic, these groups don't generally telemarket, send out direct mail, or do on-site visits.

Instead, they grow principally by buying local groups.

Well, at least that's their now-current principal strategy.

However, at some point, probably within the next several years, the pace of acquisitions is going to slow down. These large symbiotic groups won't be purchasing much any longer, and, if they do, the valuations that they'll put on potential acquisition targets will likely decrease.

Of course, that's not a complete, hard and fast rule: there will be some exceptions, some add-on acquisitions.

But for the most part, the large symbiotic groups will at some point shift to growing organically, by doing exactly what the predatory groups are doing today. That is, today's large symbiotic groups will eventually become large predatory groups: They will grow only by seeking hospital contracts directly. Why buy when they can just take?

*Single Specialty vs. Multi-Specialty*

We can also segment large groups another way: single specialty versus multispecialty

For example, in the anesthesia market, North American Partners in Anesthesia, or "NAPA," is a single specialty group. They aim on growing to become, in their minds, the dominant anesthesia group in the country.

And, on the multispecialty side, there are groups such as Sheridan which is in anesthesiology, emergency medicine, neonatology and radiology. They see the future as involving hospitals, or hospital systems, that will want to contract with one source to provide services across multiple medical specialties.

*Mindset/Vision*

Now, let's look at segmentation at the large group level, one more way. This is an issue of mindset or vision in terms of how they sell into hospital systems – how they view their relationship with the hospital.

Many large groups see the relationship with hospitals as akin to one-stop shopping for multiple service lines. In other words, the focus is still patient encounters, whether within one specialty line or even within multiple specialty lines.

However, others see the notion of partnering with hospitals as involving "episodes of care" and selling into it as a whole.

And then there are others that take a slightly different twist on this: As opposed to an episode of care, they view their role akin to what those in industry might describe as supply chain management. They seek to position themselves as providing services to the patient as the patient moves through the hospital-centered system, from transportation to the hospital, to providing services in respect of physician encounters at the hospital, to post acute care, home health, hospice, rehab, long-term care facilities, skilled nursing facility services, and so on and on and on.

Now I don't mention this to suggest that you go out and buy an ambulance . . . although I like the idea of thinking big.

Instead, I mention this because underlying this is a concept that I strongly believe you need to take to heart: I strongly believe that it will not pay to simply focus on being the best whatever-your-specialty-is that you can be. Sure, you need to focus on being the best you can be . . . but not just simply on that.

Rather, those groups that succeed will view themselves as making the experience better as well as more efficacious – for patients, yes, but also for your other customers and by that I mean primarily for hospitals.

# PART TWO

## The "World" Of Other Alternatives

# CHAPTER 3

## Do Nothing Wrong

Let's move on to discuss the "world" of other alternatives, of possible strategic moves other than being acquired.

But before we start, I don't purport that my list is all inclusive. And, note that it's possible to mix and match some of these alternatives.

With that said, the first alternative is obvious. It's probably not your first or second or even third choice, but I'd be remiss if I didn't mention it.

It's that you can do nothing different. Simply keep on doing what you've always been doing.

Note, though, that doing the same thing you've been doing is not really a strategy for success. The market is changing and you need to change along with it.

# CHAPTER 4

## Step Up Your Current Game

One certain alternative that any group can take is to step up its current game.

In fact, this is a prime example of the fact that many of the alternatives set out in this book can be combined, mixed and matched: Any group, even one considering a sale, should continuously move to improve and expand and grow its business.

Essentially, groups stepping up their game intensify and focus their current operations.

So, where do you start?

*Cementing Relationships*

Work to cement your group's relationship with each facility at which it provides services. What does the facility want? What more can you do? Ask them. Create it yourself. Come to them with ways to become more efficient and effective. Get as involved as possible in the medical staff.

Take similar action in respect of all referring physicians. Make personal contacts with them outside of the facility, when they have time to talk. What is it that they want? What more can you do? Ask them. Create it yourself. Come to them with ways to become more efficient and effective.

Pursue other facilities and opportunities. In other words, this is organic growth on your group's part. Most of the national groups started with a few doctors who grew their practice organically.

Even if your group's goal isn't to become the largest in the nation or even in your state, growing your practice beyond dependence on any one facility contact or relationship is a very important strategy for your continued success: If the only reason for your group's existence is to "serve" a single hospital, once that relationship ends, your group no longer has a reason to exist.

And, directly related to that, once the hospital administrator understands that your group owes its existence to the hospital contract, you have forfeited most, if not all of your contract negotiating leverage.

*If You Are One, Stop Being A Club*

One of the most ravaging diseases afflicting hospital-based medical groups is the disease of collegiality, of running the business like a club. Clubs consist of individuals, individuals who remain members only for so long as it benefits them personally.

In the medical group context, this results in groups that, although they bill and collect centrally (or, if they don't, they should!), are really operated in order to serve as a pass though of the funds produced by the individual physicians. In this sense, they are actually a slightly disguised expense sharing arrangement, not a true business.

Immediately work to restructure your financial operation so that the group can build and bank the capital necessary to advance, and invest in, the group's interests, no matter what those may be.

In like fashion, these groups generally run on a consensus basis. Or, they have an unwieldy board of directors: twenty members instead of three or five. Reorganize. Now!

Whether the group is set up legally as a corporation, a partnership, or some other locally authorized variant, adopt a corporate type structure with a small board or management committee charged with setting overall strategy and policy, and with a tight set of officers charged with carrying out that policy, and with making day to day operational decisions.

To sum things up, set out to tighten your group's economic operation and governance structure so that the group, and not the individual, is the primary focus of the business.

Sure, the individual shareholders and partners, just as the group's employees or subcontractors, have to be incentivized and motivated, and that comes by tying into their personal self interest. But each individual's self interest must be channeled through the entity's best interests, which must be a higher priority than any or all of the individual personal interests.

*Expand*

Pursue other business opportunities, including providing services at other facilities.

In other words, just like the large groups that I discussed above, engage in your own organic growth. After all, each of the national groups started with a few doctors who grew their practice organically.

Note that your expansion doesn't have to be within your current medical specialty. Think differently: consider moving into other specialties as well.

# CHAPTER 5

## Form A Management Entity

Form a management entity to separate out the MSO (management services organization) functions of your group's business.

For now, I'll assume that your group is sophisticated enough to have its own business office and staff. I'm not necessarily including an in-house billing and collection function, which, for many groups, is not economically viable.

Instead, what I'm addressing is a group that has a business manager who oversees the group's business operations. It might also have one or more other administrative employees.

Here's how an MSO set up of the type I'm describing looks graphically.

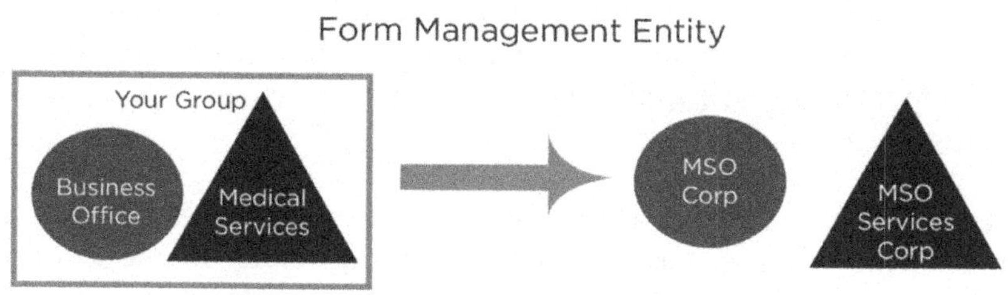

Right now the business office and the group are one and the same. Take your business operation, separate it out into a separate entity, and turn that new, separate entity into an MSO that is owned by the group's shareholders.

So, then what are the functions of that new MSO?

Well, certainly, the new MSO can continue managing your group's business. In that regard, not much would change in terms of the attention and level of service your staff provides – of course, it can always be improved!

But by splitting off the business services into a separate entity, you also put the MSO in the position to be able to sell management services to other groups, both within, and perhaps without, your specialty.

The MSO can also serve as a hub to repackage other services, such as billing and collection services which can be outsourced to another provider.

The MSO entity can operate a locum tenens service. You could utilize your current staff's overflow capacity, hire to create a locum's pool, or bring on independent practitioners as independent contractors for a particular locum's assignment.

In addition to treating this as a *tactic*, that is, seeing the MSO as simply an expansion of the group's business, you can take a more strategic view: use the MSO to create initial service relationships with a client medical group that might later expand to make the client medical group a merger or acquisition target of your own.

Additionally, placing locums at a facility allows you to gather intelligence concerning the existing relationships at that facility, perhaps opening up the facility as a future additional, permanent, service site.

And, extremely importantly, the MSO becomes a separate future salable business. Instead of simply selling your practice as a services business, the MSO is a separate entity that can be sold in a separate, or a combined, transaction. This provides additional flexibility in setting your group's strategy.

As another benefit, the existence of a truly functioning MSO operation creates an important element for some potential buyers: In the case of private equity investors new to investing either within your specialty or within the geographic region, the existence of the business operation helps to create a complete "platform." And, for some consolidators, it provides a local business base that they can take over in order to establish business operations in a new geographic area.

# CHAPTER 6

## Co-Management As An Intensification Of "Alignment" With Facilities

The next deal type we're going to discuss involves entering into a co-management agreement with a hospital as a way of intensifying the alignment between your group and the facility.

In this chapter, I'm going to show you two different "flavors" of this . . . There may be 31 flavors, who knows. *You have to understand that none of this is fixed in stone.*

That's because this is about mindset more than models: We're all guilty of looking at how others in our own industry or specialty have "*always*" done it. But how can what we do be sliced and diced, with stuff added and stuff subtracted, to get to new platforms? That's the real question.

So, with that in mind, let's get on to the first of the two "flavors" of co-management that I'll describe.

*First flavor:*

For several decades, hospital-based groups have focused on exclusive contracts to bind hospitals to a relationship and to keep competitors at bay.

But, as we all know well, there's more pressure on those relationships today. A Co-management deal is one potential solution.

The central concept of co-management is that the physician group, through an entity owned by the group alone, or through an entity owned jointly by the group and the hospital, manages a service line *with* the hospital. This differs from the relationship created under the usual exclusive contract or coverage agreement, in which the physician group provides services *to* the hospital.

Under a co-management arrangement, the management entity, and thus the physician group, is paid for management services, usually at an hourly rate, and is eligible for bonuses for meeting pre-established targets. This income is in addition to collections for professional services - those belong to the group outside of the co-management arrangement.

As an added twist, co-management structures can be built side by side with exclusive contracts. And, the existence of the management relationship, especially one in which both the group and the hospital own the management company, provides a strong business reason for the hospital to continue to renew the exclusive contract with the "partner" group.

Co-management agreements present compliance issues not present in the everyday exclusive contract or coverage agreement. They take a significant degree of initiative on the part of the group to form and, once in place, take real effort to carry out.

But the payoff can be very real in terms of improvement in patient care and improvement in the hospital's efficiency and cost structure . . . with a financial reward flowing to the physician group. These arrangements preserve independence yet *align* interests in a way that differs from the pejorative sense of that word.

Here's how a co-management structure can look graphically.

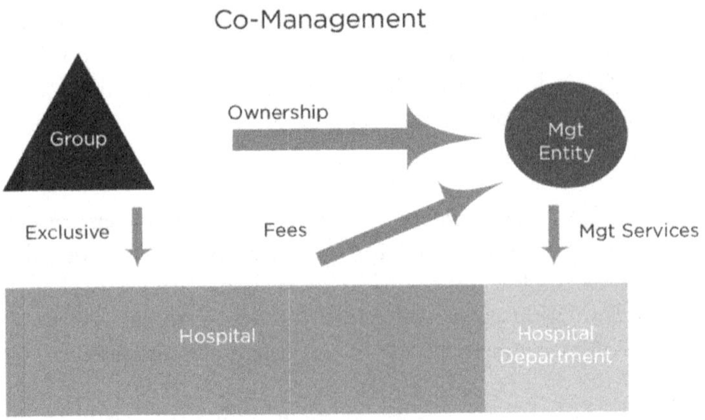


Note also how the existence of the management relationship binds the group closer to the hospital thereby extending the relationship.

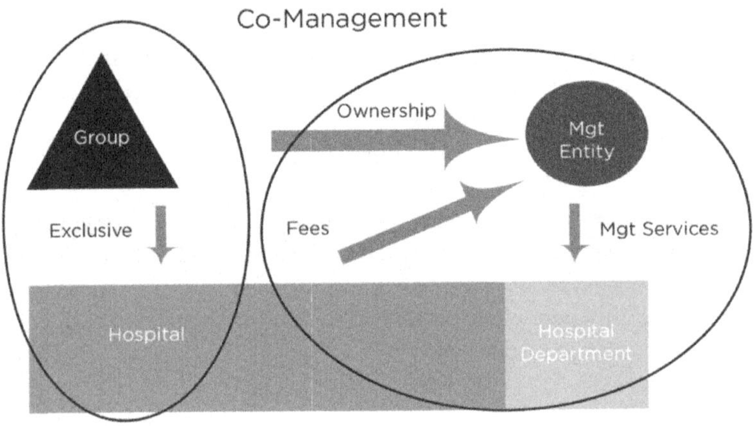

*And Now On To The Second Flavor:*

In this second form, or "flavor" as I've called it, of co-management, the hospital can be a co-owner of the management entity with you.

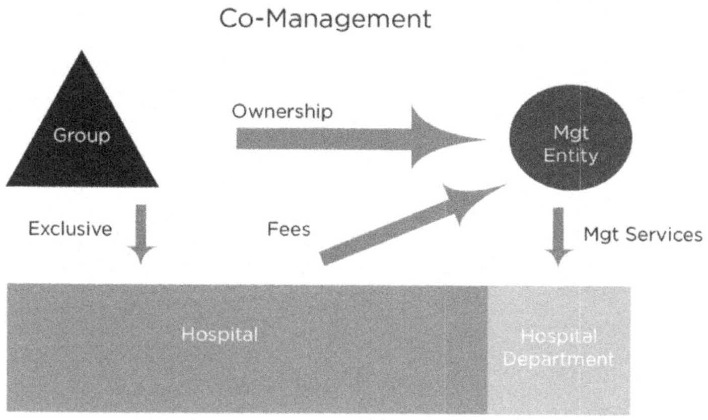


There is also a double scoop form of this second flavor: Form a joint venture to sell both management services and professional services.

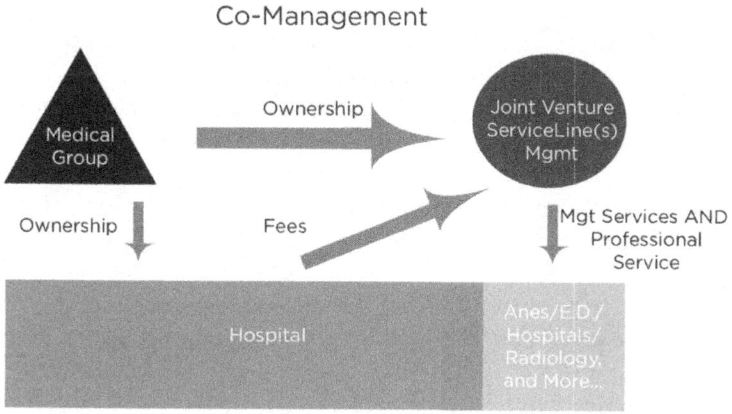

# CHAPTER 7

## But How?

When working with clients on their strategic future, it's at this point in the process that I usually see the worried look on their faces.

Not all the time, mind you. But often.

It's caused by the gap, mostly in their thinking, between where they are and where they want to be. Specifically, they wonder how in heck they can pull off stepping up their own game or creating a management entity.

So, before going to further to discuss ventures that involve partnering in one form or another with a third party, let's take a look at *how* you would begin to pursue those efforts.

First, very obviously from the outside but somehow and often invisible from the position of those within the group, the group can do it on its own.

In other words, you can hire staff or, if you already have *some* non-professional staff, you can grow it: Allow your in-house administrator to use the full range of his or her expertise. Your existing business operation can be grown into an engine of growth.

And you can also buy expertise from consultants and other experts as needed. For example, from me. (I am not shy!) Or, from your group's current billing service or from another one. Or, from some management entity, whether it brands itself as an MSO or simply as a services provider.

The "why" you want to do this, in other words, your strategy and your goals, is what's important. The "how" you'll do it is a detail.

# CHAPTER 8

## Align With An MSO

This alternative is very, very different from the notion, discussed above, of forming your own management services organization, or MSO.

Instead of developing your group's own business structure to provide management services to other groups, this alternative has your group outsourcing some or all of its management role to a third party MSO.

Generally, although there's no rule that requires that it always be true, MSOs charge anesthesia groups a fee based on a percentage of collections – this is the same general model employed by billing and collection services.

Note also that the menu of services can vary broadly among MSOs. Some incorporate the billing and collection function, others don't. Some actively seek out business opportunities for their clients, others don't (or say that they do, but don't). And so on.

Here, graphically, is what contracting with an MSO generally looks like.

Co-Management

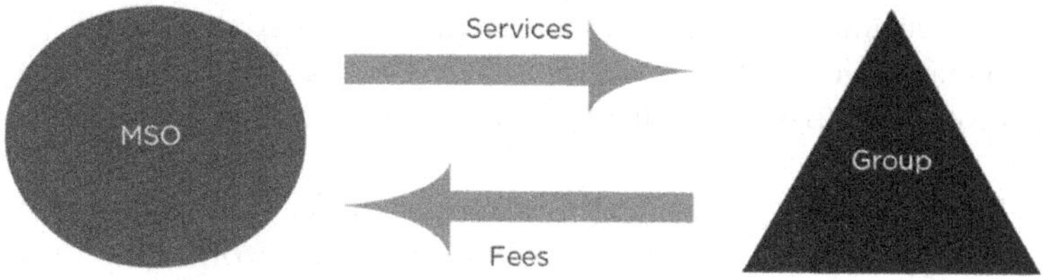


For me, the question is, "Why?" Why align with an MSO? What's in it for you?

Note that the issue of obtaining business management services from an MSO is distinct from obtaining billing and collection services from a traditional sort of hospital-based third party billing service.

Generally, the decision to obtain services from a third party MSO is driven by a group's lack of a business infrastructure.

If your group has a business infrastructure, whether one comprised of the efforts of group members who take an active role in business or, preferably, through management staff working at the direction of group leadership, especially an infrastructure that that can be grown, then what's the draw in paying a third party for those services?

If your group doesn't have a business infrastructure, then it should start, right now, to develop one.

Many MSOs tout that they are an alternative for their clients to "joining" a national group. It may technically be an alternative (so is just going out of business) but often it's difficult to understand the reasoning.

Some MSOs are viable alternatives to the formation of a regional or national group; they use their structure to avoid the trap of prohibitions on the corporate practice of medicine in some or all of the states in which they do business.

And, of course, I haven't seen every MSO and some might offer tremendous advantages – so at a minimum, conduct a full due diligence review prior to entering into any contract.

Unfortunately, in my experience, MSOs are not particularly great at selling their client's services into new sites. And, if they could pull that off, how, after all, can they deal with the conflict of growing each of their client's businesses – that is, unless they've got only one client in each region, and even that depends on a shared vision of the region within which promoting any particular client group's business will be restricted.

Instead, MSOs are generally business vehicles the owners of which are attempting to build up and then sell for their own profit – there's absolutely nothing wrong with that. But query then whether there should be a "reverse fee?" Should your group receive an interest in the MSO because by "aligning" with, your group is likely building its value more than you are building your own?

On the other hand, despite these defects, after a thorough inquiry, if you determine that you are going to align with an MSO, then what kind of MSO would you align with?

We can segment MSOs several ways.

For example, we can segment them by whether they're active in a single medical specialty or in multiple medical specialties.

And, we can segment them by whether they work on the physician side, only, or whether they court hospital business to "manage" other physicians. The pitch made by those MSOs on the hospital side is something akin to "hospital, hire us and put us in a position such that the local group is required to use our services." Or, even, "hospital use our services in connection with forcing independent physicians into hospital employment."

Also, you need to question what you're really going to be getting from the MSO relationship.

Is the MSO simply a billing service with an add on fee for "management services?" Is the MSO repackaging billing services provided by an outside vendor with an additional fee tacked on? Can those same management services be obtained in reverse: from a billing service that doesn't masquerade as an MSO for it's usual fee plus a reduced add on fee for the management services?

Watch out for a Promise – Delivery Gap™. If they say that they'll grow your business, ask how, exactly, they will do it. They can't approach multiple facilities as if they are a group. On the legal side, depending on your state, there are corporate practice of medicine problems. On the business side, if they work with multiple groups, why do you think that they will be expanding your opportunities and not those of some other group?

And, ponder this: Are you going to give up so much control to an MSO that it's as if you've been sold, just without the purchase price?

The bottom line: There may be advantages provided to you by a particular MSO. On the other hand, it may not be of any value to you – or worse. So, adopt an approach analogous to that of carpentry: measure twice, cut once.

# CHAPTER 9

## Merger

Let's move on to another structure, one that doesn't require that you pay cash: Merger.

When I use the term "merger," I primarily mean a deal in which your group essentially acquires another group by way of merging it into yours.

Of course, if you're interested in a variant, your group and another group could form a completely new entity and each abandon its current legal form, merging into the new entity. At the conclusion of that arrangement, the old groups' respective owners would become the owners of the new entity. In fact, we'll look at that last model at the end of this chapter.

But to begin, let's look at the notion of using a merger tactic to acquire another group.

The first step is to identify and pursue the merger partner.

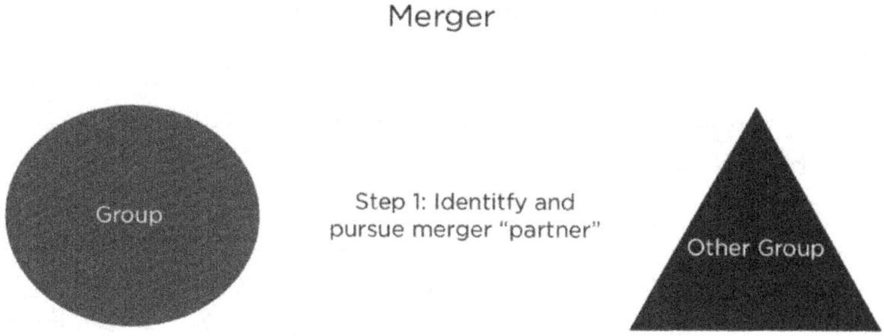


Note that, although it's well outside the scope of this book, the elements that make a successful merger go beyond the obvious financial considerations. Elements such as group culture, governance style, compensation expectations, among many others, play an important role in the long term viability of a merger deal.

Then, as the second step, trade equity interests in your group to the owners of the merger partner in exchange for their interests in that entity.

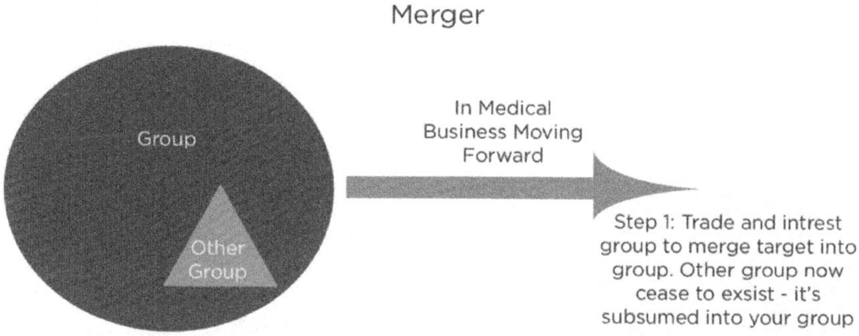


The other group now ceases to exist – it's subsumed into your group. Then if you so wish, "rinse and repeat," growing your group through subsequent merger transactions.

Using a merger strategy, you can aggregate to acquire the right groups – the right people, the right culture, the right reimbursement – to become a larger player.

As a result, you can seek multi-hospital system agreements and potentially negotiate higher reimbursement from payors due to your size and clout. This becomes an engine for more growth.

Or you can take that larger, merged entity and, with more mass, sell it in the future at, potentially, a higher valuation.

And, as mentioned above, your group and another group (or multiple other groups) can form a completely new entity. Each of the existing group entities is abandoned. Your group's owners and the owners of the other group or groups then become owners of the new entity.

This, too is generally a "no cash exchanges hands" kind of deal.

Essentially, it's "partnering up" with someone else. The partnership could, like any of the deal partners, be single specialty or multispecialty.

Here, graphically, is an example of how one such structure could be set up. There are other variants of this model using other forms of legal structure and other methods of creating the new, jointly owned "partnership."

At "Time 1," (see the image, below) there's your group, depicted by the green circle, and an existing partnership model group.

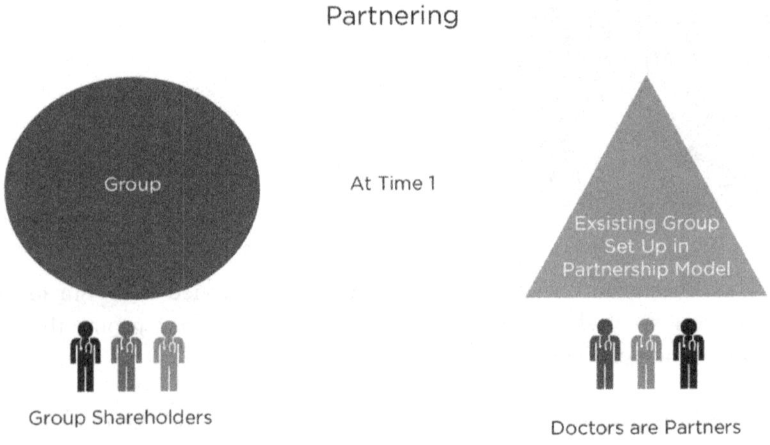

At "Time 2," your existing group liquidates. The doctors who were formerly the owners of your group now become additional owners of partnership entity. (Of course, each should do so a via limited liability vehicle, such as a professional corporation).

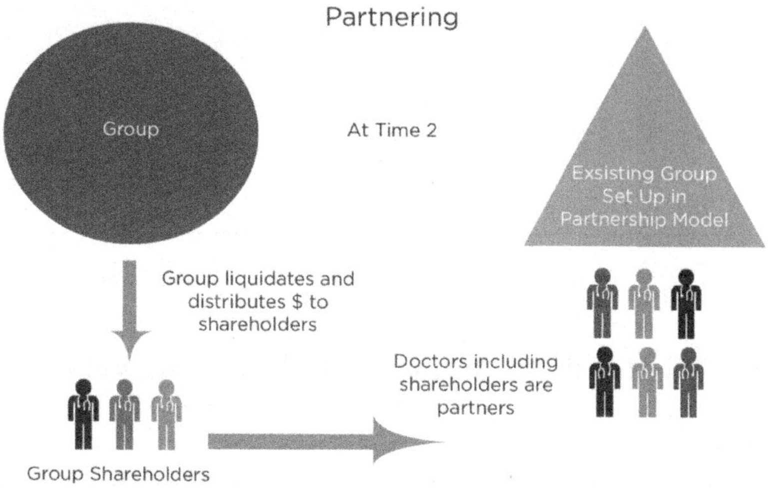


Finally, note that your group could be the sponsor of a partnership model as an alternative to acquiring other groups or merging with them. This is another way of bulking up for significance in the market and for a potential later sale.

# CHAPTER 10

## Hybrid Model: An Alliance or Joint Venture Vehicle

Before addressing the much larger issue of an acquisition, let's have a very quick look at a final alternative structure, a hybrid that I call an alliance or joint venture vehicle.

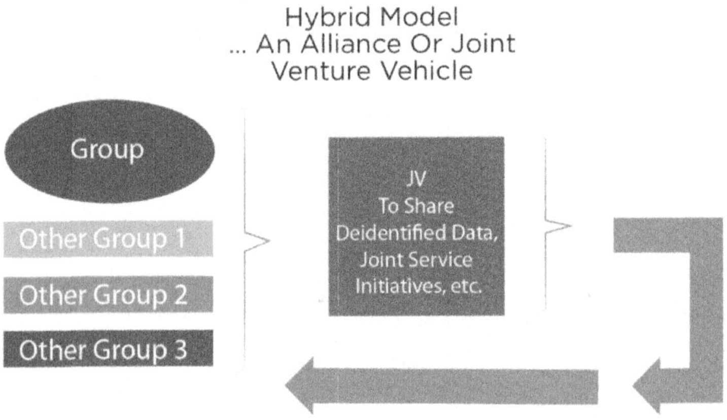


This is a cooperative venture. In it, each group continues to operate on its own, but now under the umbrella of the alliance.

Note that the alliance structure shown is not an MSO. There's no requirement that the alliance vehicle provide services back to the constituent entities and there's no requirement that the alliance members pay the alliance itself for any services.

That said, there's no reason that the alliance can't include an MSO function as an add-on component in order to sell services to the constituent members and, perhaps, to third parties as well, with the profit going back to support the joint venture entity's operations

For example, your group could, together with another group or, preferably a number of other groups, local or distant, form an alliance or joint venture to provide the verisimilitude of size.

Members of the joint venture alliance can then jointly cooperate in various initiatives for their own, as well as mutual, benefit. For example, they could share and use de-identified patient data for quality improvement. They can jointly develop programs and service initiatives to carry out on their own at their service locations or even jointly on a broader, public relations scale.

It's even possible that the alliance can develop some cross coverage arrangements or a locums type service, make use of some shared technology, and so on.

# PART THREE

## Acquisitions

# CHAPTER 11

## Acquisition Basics

There are many ways to structure an actual acquisition.

In general, however, an acquisition can be structured as a sale of stock or as sale of assets. Here, in the illustration below, is a very simple generalized model showing how this would work in practice. The group is essentially selling to a captive entity owned by the acquirer. That entity is the new practice owner.

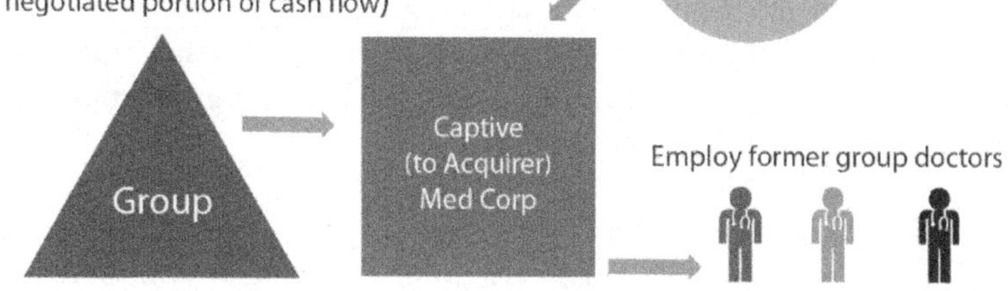

Let me show you a variant, another generalized model.

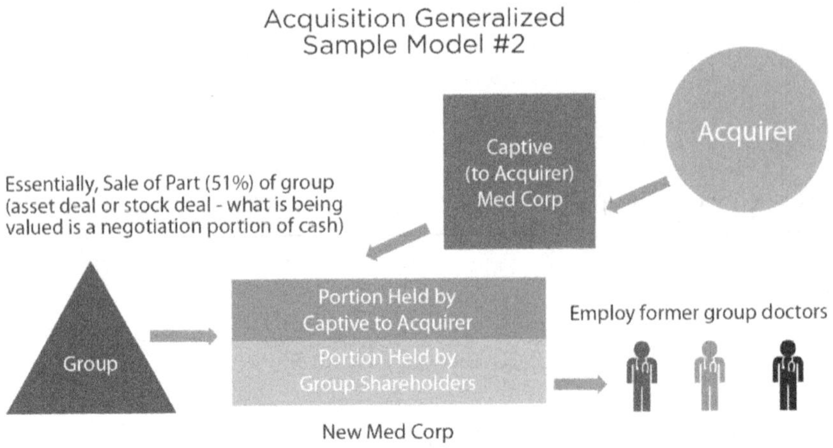


In the second, general example, the resulting new practice entity is jointly owned.

So in either of these generalized models, other than, say for a radiology group that has imaging equipment that has value, all that most groups actually have to sell is a portion of their cash flow.

I say "a portion," because it would be extremely rare that a buyer would allow you to sell more than what is really your profit, that is, that amount above your market level salaries so that the physicians don't quit . . . so that the acquired group can continue to recruit and retain.

I want you to understand that this type of acquisition is somewhat different from selling, say, a manufacturing business in which there are hard assets involved. As opposed to a manufacturing business, which has fixed assets, inventory, and the like, unless a hospital-based group has significant assets, all it has to sell is its cash flow.

So, for example, if, and I'm just playing with numbers here, a hypothetical group sold $5,000,000 of annual cash flow (and there are limits on what can really be sold as almost any buyer would want to leave enough cash flow in the group to pay market salaries) and if the group received a 7 times multiple, there'd be a value of $35,000,000.

In essence, the buyer in this example is recouping (ignoring for now the concept of interest and the difference between ordinary income and capital gains tax rates) its money over 7 years. But, of course, the deal keeps on running *ad infinitum.*

So, what the group is really doing is selling future earnings and shifting the risk that over the "multiples term," here there being a 7 times multiple, or 7 years, that an amount equivalent to the purchase price will fail to come in: for example, the risk that their exclusive contract will be terminated or that payor rates will precipitously drop.

Of course, there's also the issue of what amount of income will be guaranteed as compensation to the selling physicians, and for how long. In other words, when can their compensation be cut to even lower levels? And, after the guaranty burns off, if the hospital contract is lost, the selling physicians will be looking for new jobs.

Note here, too, that the actual acquirer, the actual employer, is highly unlikely to be a big entity; rather, it's often the case that it will be a local company, a "NewCo," set up to do the acquisition. How financially stable is it and what guaranties can be had from its parent?

You can readily see that, all other things being the same, physicians closer to retirement age or who are planning on leaving the group in a few years will tend to be far more supportive of an acquisition deal than those who have many more years of practice.

That's because those near retirement or departure will collect a chunk of cash now and not be around for too many years, if any, at reduced pay. On the other hand, the younger docs will be around at lower salaries for a long period of time.

Needless to say, non-shareholders and those not yet even recruited don't have a say in the matter, at least in the corporate or partnership sense: They may, however, vote with their feet or, depending upon what representations were made to them of future partnership, with a lawsuit.

*Are You Really A Seller?*

Query whether if you're the group being acquired, are you actually a seller or is it that you're really the buyer?

In other words, are the selling shareholders or partners actually "buying" cash up front in return for reduced earnings long term?

It should quickly become apparent that, unlike the sale of a hypothetical manufacturing company in which the owner sells for millions and moves on, having received his or her profit from the sale of the business, in a hospital-based group acquisition deal, it's almost a certainty that physicians staying with the group for a number of years exceeding the multiple will have self financed the entire purchase price and, following that, will likely earn less as the result of having made the sale. They will, in essence, be paying the buyer for their jobs.

What's the best way to "spend" that reduction in earnings? Is it to fund the cash up front or is it to fund the expansion of your business as an alternative to selling your group?

Now, in all fairness, those in favor of selling also see a shifting of risk – the sellers will receive the purchase price which is essentially an advance of future earnings, but if it's all received now, then it's protected, protected from what would happen if it couldn't be earned because the group's exclusive contract is terminated or payor rates drop within the multiples period.

That notion of protection is true to some degree. What's been shifted is timing – money is being received up front and essentially paid back over the following years of likely lower compensated employment. When those "lines" cross, the risk is done shifting in the selling physicians' favor. After that, as long as the contractual relationship between the group and the facility stays in place, the sellers will continue to "shift" funds back to the buyer, as discussed above.

But remember, also, for those lump sum dollars to have value as protection for the future, they must be invested in a way that both protects the principal and results in a rate of growth that meets or exceeds the return that the selling physicians would receive under the alternative scenario: for example, no sale and a continued contract which puts more money into their pockets.

There are other factors in favor of a sale to the *right* buyer.

For example, if the buyer has, or can obtain, much more favorable payor contracts than the selling group, or has a much better handle on expenses, some or all of the decrease in compensation as a result of the sale might be replaced by higher income at the group level.

The devil is clearly in the details: If your group's income were significantly higher than the market to begin with, even after a sale, the individual former owners would likely find themselves with compensation within the bounds of the "normal" market range. In other words, much less than before but at so-called market. Consider, though, that if that level is truly market, there would be little pressure on the new owner to later allow per physician income to drift upwards.

As a final example of the factors leading to sale, some sellers seek an exit from local ownership because they believe that their group has peaked, or worse. They have no strategy for the future or have no faith in the strategy that they have.

As a result, they believe that combining with a buyer will provide them with the benefit of a road map. In some cases, sellers take part of the purchase consideration in cash and part in equity in the buyer, seeking to, they hope, realize even more value in the future when (and if) that equity piece becomes more valuable.

# Chapter 12

## Thoughts On Acquirers

If a group is going to sell, then certainly one of the essential questions is "sell to whom?"

It's possible to segment potential acquisition partners, that is, buyers, a number of ways. I'll go through some of those ways in this chapter. But be aware that there are other ways to group buyers, too.

*In The Medical Business vs. In The Investment (In Medical Business) Business*

Certainly, one of the easiest ways to segment buyers is to look at those which are actually in the business of running a large medical group.

Of course, there's no guaranty that those buyers, even the ones that are publicly held, won't be acquired by another entity at some point in the future.

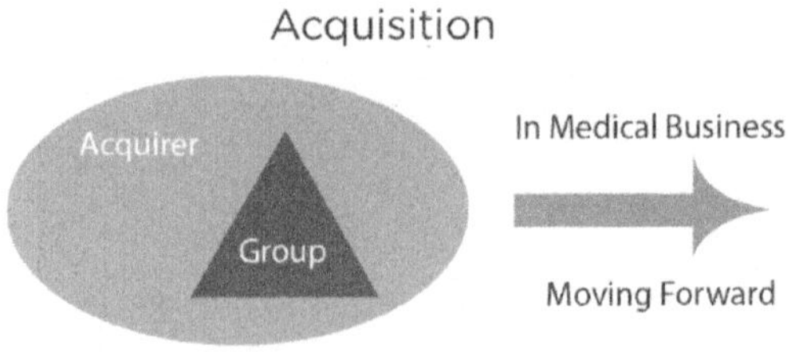


And, on the other hand, you have deals with private equity folks who see an investment in medical groups as a good one and therefore buy the business with a goal to exit via sale or public offering in 3 to 5 to 8 years.

They are not themselves in the medical business, they're in the investment business and they're investing *their investors'* funds to purchase you

So we have a purchase in 2015 and a sale to someone else in 2018 or 2020. These are money partners, not medical practice partners. There's nothing inherently wrong about this; these buyers are totally upfront with you about this. That's their business. If you were a bakery and bakeries were hot investments, they'd buy and flip you, too.

The question then is whether you want to be in business with, no, actually, do you want to work for, someone who's going to be a partner (and I use that word very loosely) for a potentially long run or for the time that it takes to flip the business as an exit strategy? Does your answer change if you continue to own a small piece of the business that will be flipped, in other words, if you took a part of your sale consideration in the form of an equity interest in the buyer?

*Single Specialty vs. Multi-Specialty*

We can also segment potential acquisition partners into those pursuing a single specialty model versus those buyers developing a multi-specialty platform.

No matter whether a group is acquired or not, your continued ability to practice at the location or locations served by your group now, whether through that group or through the group that acquires your group, is dependent upon the continuation of the contract at your facility or facilities. Accordingly, post sale, the buyer's strategy, single specialty or multi-specialty, may have an impact on the continuation of your contract.

It's not as if you are taking a job with an employer that, if they lose the contract at one or more of your facilities, will seamlessly transfer you to some other job site. Maybe they will have an opening somewhere, maybe not. And, it's not likely that an actual national group is going to employ you; it will most likely be a pop-up entity under their control that makes the acquisition and then employs you.

*Encounter vs. Supply Chain*

If we really want to get deep into the inner workings of buyers, we can also segment potential acquisition partners into those focused on selling services related to an encounter versus those looking at the larger picture of selling to manage the patient along a "supply chain," as we discussed earlier.

These are issues of concept, and of strategy.

So, very roughly, the graphic below shows an encounter type outlook. Note that one subset of an encounter strategy sells to multiple hospitals. Another subset targets hospital chains, bypassing single or even multiple hospital contracts to try to get a whole system or at least a large region of a system into a contract.

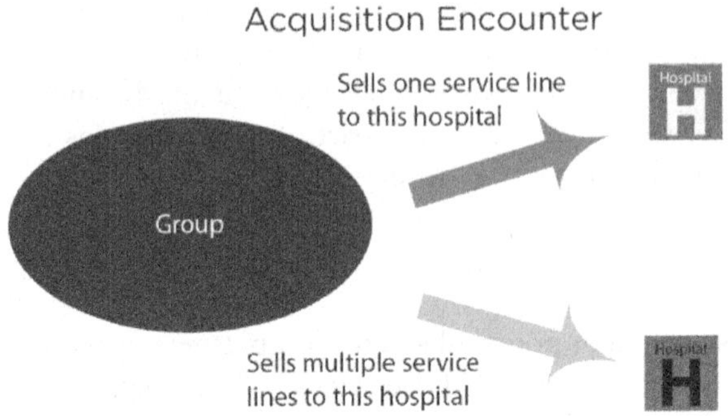


And, again, very roughly, here's a "supply chain" outlook.

Instead of focusing on one or several discrete services, the strategy is to contract to provide all of a large menu of patient-side services from pre-admission to post-discharge care.

Note that this strategy can be deployed in respect of a single hospital or to an entire hospital system or region of a system.

Acquisition "Supply Chain"

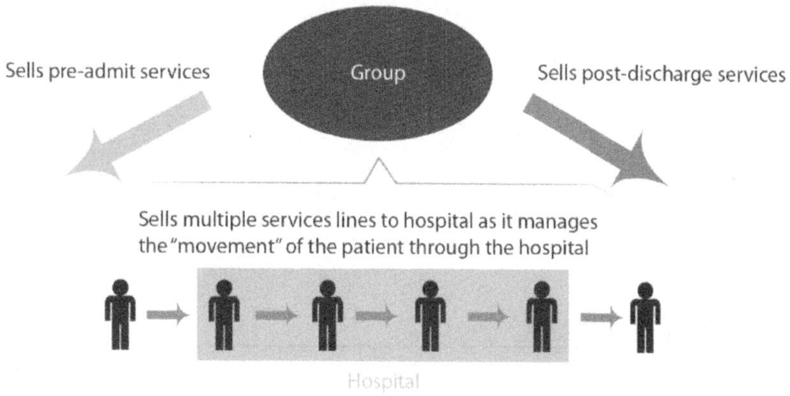


*By Staffing Model*

We can also segment buyers by their staffing model.

Certainly, within anesthesiology, this means those that focus on a care team model, an all M.D. model, or even a model in which M.D.s and CRNAs are working independently side by side.

*By Growth Model*

We can also segment acquirers by their growth model.

Some very active acquirers as of the time of this writing focus on growth by acquisition. In other words, they are growing their business by buying local groups.

On the other hand, other acquirers are not only purchasing local groups, they are responding to RFPs and pitching their services directly to facilities at the same time.

# PART FOUR

## Thought Tools For Use In Analysis Of Options

# CHAPTER 13

## Thought Tools

I'd like to wind our discussion down by giving you some thought tools to frame the issues in your analysis of potential mergers, acquisitions and alternatives.

The following aren't in any particular order.

Imagine it's 5 years from now. Where are you, both personally and professionally?

The only way that this question will be valuable is that you must also think what's best for the group, not simply what's best for you, individually.

What's your ability to manage the growth of your group from within?

Are you willing to invest in your group's future? You can't be cheap – you'll hinder your future.

***

There will always be predatory groups competing for your facility contracts. That's the case whether you sell the group or run your own group.

---

Groups that are large today have either grown from an initial practice with a real business operation . . . or they have grown by having one provided to it by a money partner, the trade off being that that partner is in the position to take some or all of the growth.

The private equity firms are looking to triple or better their money . . . they certainly see a bright future in terms of the value of an acquired group. They are taking that upside, or most of it.

Why do they see the future so bright when others (you?) see it so dark?

---

Do you want to control your practice?

Are you wiling to give it up for $X of value?

What are you really paying (giving up) in potential dollars to get that $X of value?

---

If you sell and have a guaranty for Y years, what's your exit plan after that period?

---

What are you looking for in an acquisition partner? Short term relationship or a long term one?

---

Are you willing to place a cap, or, at best, a governor, on your future earnings?

---

Note that there's no requirement of a binary decision, of a single choice.

Instead it is a moving loop of concurrent options.

---

There's no right answer and no wrong answer. No magic bullet.

But remember that . . .

Your practice will continue to be impacted by disruptive change in the healthcare market.

You have all the excuses as to why you're a victim of disruption. But you also have all the opportunity of disruption that you can use. So, it boils down to your choice.

# SPECIAL FREE GIFT FROM THE AUTHOR

You're invited to obtain a free copy of the webinar recording *Medical Group Mergers And Acquisitions And Alternatives*, a $397 value.

To obtain your copy, without charge, go to the following site, now: www.advisorylawgroup.com/mergersgiveaway.html

# FREE BOOK DOWNLOAD

## Directions: Clarity for Medical Group Leaders

The healthcare market is changing rapidly, bringing new sets of problems.

How can you find a solution, how can you engage in the right development of strategy, and how can you to plan your, or your group's, future without tools to help clarify your thinking?

*Directions* is a collection of thoughts as thinking tools, each intended to instruct, inform, and even more so, cause you to give pause to instruct and inform yourself.

Go to www.advisorylawgroup.com/blogbookdownload.html now to download your free copy.

# KNOWLEDGE PRODUCTS

## Breaking News On Kickbacks: The Latest On The Company Model

The recording of Mark F. Weiss' webinar Breaking News On Kickbacks: The Latest On The Company Model. As the healthcare economy becomes more strained, the pace of illegal kickback activity has increased. Join Mark F. Weiss, attorney for the Requestor of OIG Advisory Opinion 13-15, to learn the absolute latest on the so-called Company Model.

Audio Version $279
Video Version $379
Audio and Video Version $379

To purchase Breaking News On Kickbacks: The Latest On The Company Model go to www.advisorylawgroup.com/knowledgeproducts.html

## Double Indemnity: Putting Yourself At Risk For Millions – The Interplay Between Insurance And Indemnification Provisions In Your Hospital And Physician Contracts

They may look like boilerplate, but your feet might be in the boiler's fire if you haven't properly thought through the impact and interplay of the indemnification and insurance provisions in your contracts with hospitals and with providers.

Audio Version $129
Video Version $179
Video and Audio Versions $179

To purchase **Double Indemnity: Putting Yourself At Risk For Millions – The Interplay Between Insurance And Indemnification Provisions In Your Hospital And Physician Contracts** go to www.advisorylawgroup.com/knowledgeproducts.html

## Disruptive Strategies In Healthcare: Designing Them And Dealing With Them

Believing that the future of the business of healthcare will be a projection of, or incremental improvement over, today's reality is a fool's game.

Although predicting the specifics of the future is impossible, it's certain to involve disruptive strategies. Think, for example, of the disruption to the private practice of medicine resulting from the blossoming hospital-centric worldview. But are you aware of the disruptive strategies aimed at shattering that worldview?

There are only two sides to the healthcare coin: figure out a way to disrupt the current practice model or figure out how to deal with someone else's disruption.

By purchasing you'll understand the role of disruption in healthcare, you'll learn of disruptive events currently on the horizon, you'll learn key elements in designing disruptive strategies and you'll understand how best to protect your practice from someone else's disruption.

Audio Version $107
Video Version $197
Audio and Video Version $197

To purchase **Disruptive Strategies In Healthcare: Designing Them And Dealing With Them** go to
www.advisorylawgroup.com/knowledgeproducts.html

## Why Your Medical Group Needs A New Contracting Strategy

No matter your political bent, there's no doubt that society is becoming increasingly affected by "we" think, from concepts of shared sacrifice, to paying your fair share, to "giving back."

These notions of community and cooperation present an advantage to local medical groups in fighting off the onslaught of outside competitors.

But that advantage will be lost unless medical groups adopt a contracting strategy that harmonizes with the growing societal trends.

When you watch or listen to this thirty-minute webinar, you'll learn:

- The major general societal trends.
- How those trends impact medical group relationships.
- How those trends impact medical group facility contracting.
- Why having a strategy that ties into those trends provides you with an essential advantage.

Audio Version $97
Video Version $129
Video and Audio Versions

To purchase **Why Your Medical Group Needs A New Contracting Strategy**
go to www.advisorylawgroup.com/knowledgeproducts.html

## Reverse Engineering A National Takeover Of Your Facility Contract

Like a neutron bomb, national or large regional groups wants to take over your facility contract, vaporize your group, and cherry-pick your desirable assets: your physicians and other providers.

By understanding their approach, you'll drastically increase your group's chances for survival.

In the approximately 45 minutes of this recording of an ALG Webinar, you'll learn:

The strategies and tactics national groups use to approach hospitals.
What they are saying about you.
What you can do proactively to inoculate your group against their approach.
Other tools for protecting your group from planned contractual annihilation.

Audio recording: $397
Complete video of webinar: $497
Audio recording and complete video: $497

To purchase **Reverse Engineering A National Takeover Of Your Facility Contract**
go to www.advisorylawgroup.com/knowledgeproducts.html

## How To Deal With RFPs For Physician Services

More and more hospitals are disrupting their relationships with hospital-based and office-based physicians.

The favored tool? The request for proposal, commonly known as an "RFP."

How can an RFP be avoided?

Do you respond?

How do you respond?

How can the rules be bent?

These are among the issues discussed in this recording of an ALG Webinar. You'll receive practical and actionable information for your group's immediate application.

After viewing the recording or listening to the audio of this ALG Webinar, you'll have:

- An understanding of the three types of RFPs
- Knowledge of the strategies and tactics used to avoid RFPs
- Awareness of the major defect in the RFP process
- Knowledge of strategies and tactics used to respond to RFPs
- An understanding of the importance of a strategy aimed outside of the RFP process itself

Purchase How to Deal with RFPs for Physician Services now:

Audio recording: $207
Complete video of webinar: $297
Audio recording and complete video: $297

To purchase **How to Deal With RFPs For Physician Services** go to www.advisorylawgroup.com/knowledgeproducts.html

Made in the USA
Monee, IL
04 November 2026

67387904R00046